Solution to Prevent Death

Ideas & Techniques for Living a Long, Healthy, and Meaningful Life

By

Sarah P. Jackson

Table of Content

Introduction

Preventing premature death is an objective that everyone should pursue. While we can do a few things to increase our chances of living a long and healthy life, we cannot control every factor that could cause early death. We can lower our risk of developing chronic diseases and other health conditions resulting in premature death by adopting lifestyle choices promoting physical and mental health.

In this guide, we'll look at various ways to avoid death before it happens. We will talk about how important it is to eat a healthy diet, exercise frequently, avoid high-risk behaviors, get enough sleep, manage stress, and get regular medical checkups. You can take charge of your health and well-being with the help of these suggestions, increasing your chances of living a long and fulfilling life. Therefore, let's begin!

The significance of avoiding death before it is necessary cannot be overstated.

If we pass away too soon, we will miss out on the many experiences and relationships that make life worthwhile and the chance to live a full and content life. It also significantly impacts those we leave behind, such as loved ones and friends.

Poor lifestyle choices, environmental factors, and genetic predispositions all have the potential to contribute to premature death. By avoiding these things, we can lower our risk of dying too soon and increase our chances of living a longer and healthier life.

In addition, premature death can have a significant financial impact on the affected person's and their family's quality of life, as well as an increase in healthcare costs and lost productivity. As a result, people and society benefit from avoiding premature death.

In conclusion, avoiding harm is crucial for our health, those we care about, and the health of society at large. Premature death. It is a goal that deserves our full attention, and we should do everything in our power to preserve our health and extend our lives.

Several general principles that can assist us in maintaining our health and avoiding premature death exist.

These are some:

Avoiding processed and high-sugar foods while maintaining a healthy diet rich in fruits, vegetables, lean proteins, and whole grains.

At least 30 minutes a day, five days a week, of regular physical activity, such as walking, running, biking, or swimming.

Avoiding high-risk behaviors like smoking, drinking too much alcohol, and using drugs.

Getting the recommended seven to nine hours of sleep each night for adults.

Utilizing techniques like mindfulness, meditation, or exercises in deep breathing to manage stress.

Keeping up with regular medical examinations, including screenings for chronic conditions like diabetes, heart disease, and cancer.

Maintaining a healthy weight through regular physical activity and a well-balanced diet.

By adhering to these general principles, we can support our overall health and lower our risk of developing chronic diseases that could result in premature death. Additionally, these principles encourage good mental and physical health, which can enhance our quality of life and assist us in living lives that are both longer and more satisfying.

Chapter 1

Maintain a Healthy Diet

Preventing premature death requires a healthy diet. A well-balanced diet can help lower the risk of chronic diseases like diabetes, cancer, and heart disease. To maintain a healthy diet, follow these guidelines:

Eat various vegetables and fruits: Vitamins, minerals, and antioxidants in these foods aid in disease prevention. Aim for a daily intake of at least five fruits and vegetables.

Whole grains are best: Whole grains are an excellent source of dietary fiber and other essential nutrients. Whole-grain products like brown rice and bread should be your go-to choices.

Consume lean proteins: Choose protein from beans, lentils, chicken, fish, and other lean sources. Saturated fat, which can raise cholesterol levels and the risk of heart disease, is lower in these foods.

Eat foods that are processed and high in sugar: These foods frequently have a lot of calories, bad fats, and added sugars, making you gain weight and more likely to get chronic diseases.

Reduce your alcohol intake: Overindulging in alcohol consumption has been linked to an increased risk of liver disease, certain types of cancer, and other health issues. Aim for one drink daily for women and no more than two for men.

By adhering to these dietary guidelines, we can support our overall health and lower our risk of developing chronic diseases that could result in premature death. Furthermore, a solid eating routine can advance great physical and psychological well-being, which can improve our personal satisfaction and help us live longer and more satisfying lives.

Significance of a fair eating regimen

A fair eating regimen is significant because it gives us the supplements our body needs to work appropriately. It is necessary for promoting longevity, preventing chronic diseases, and maintaining good health. Here are a few justifications for why a reasonable eating routine is significant:

Contains vital nutrients: All of the essential nutrients our bodies require, including carbohydrates, proteins, fats, vitamins, and minerals, can be found in a well-balanced diet. Our body's growth, repair, and maintenance depend on these nutrients.

Assists in preventing chronic diseases: Chronic diseases like diabetes, some cancers, and heart disease can all be avoided with a well-balanced diet low in sodium, saturated and trans fats, cholesterol, and other nutrients.

Helps maintain a healthy weight: Maintaining a healthy weight, which can lower the risk of chronic diseases and improve overall health, can be made easier with a well-balanced diet high in fruits, vegetables, whole grains, and lean proteins.

Boosts one's energy: A reasonable eating routine that incorporates complex carbs, like entire grains, can give supported energy for the day, assisting us with feeling more ready and centered.

Bolsters mental well-being: Omega-3-rich foods like nuts, fish, and seeds can support brain function and lower the risk of depression and other mental health conditions when part of a well-balanced diet.

In conclusion, eating a well-balanced diet is important for staying healthy, avoiding chronic diseases, and increasing longevity. We can support our overall health and lower our risk of premature death by consuming various healthy foods and avoiding those high in sodium, sugar, and unhealthy fats.

Foods that are processed and high in sugar should be avoided at all costs

If you want to keep a healthy diet and lower your risk of dying too soon. These foods often have a lot of calories, bad fats, and added sugars, making you gain weight and more likely to get chronic diseases. Here are a few ways to keep away from handled and high-sugar food varieties:

Read labels on food: Look for foods that don't have many added sugars, sodium, or bad fats. Products with long lists of ingredients that are hard to identify should be avoided.

Limit sweet beverages: Energy drinks, fruit juices, and soft drinks typically have a lot of sugar and calories. Instead, select water or beverages without added sugar.

Whole foods are best: Fruits, vegetables, whole grains, and lean proteins are examples of whole foods that are less processed and contain more nutrients than processed foods.

Avoid cheap food: Fast food typically contains a lot of sodium, unhealthy fats, and calories. Salads, grilled chicken, and roasted vegetables are all healthier options.

Homemade meals: You can control the ingredients and avoid harmful additives when you cook at home. Make healthier choices and save time by preparing meals in advance.

By avoiding processed and high-sugar foods, we can support our overall health and lower our risk of developing chronic diseases that could result in premature death. Additionally, eating a diet high in whole foods and low in added sugars can help us live longer and more meaningful lives by improving our physical and mental health.

Eat a lot of fruits and vegetables

Eating many fruits and vegetables is important for keeping a healthy diet and lowering your risk of dying too soon. Vitamins, minerals, fiber, and antioxidants in fruits and vegetables aid in disease prevention. Eat a lot of fruits and vegetables by following these guidelines:

Attempt variety: Eating various fruits and vegetables can provide a wide range of nutrients and flavors. Every day, try to eat fruits and vegetables of various colors and varieties.

Choose produce still in season: Compared to canned or frozen produce, fresh produce typically has more nutrients and is often more flavorful. Choosing produce that is in season can also help cut costs.

Include vegetables and fruits in your meals and snacks: Add cut foods grown from the ground to plates of mixed greens, sandwiches, and wraps. Consume fresh vegetables and fruits for snacks or blend them into smoothies.

Healthy ways to prepare vegetables include steaming, dishing, or barbecuing vegetables instead of searing them. Instead of salt, use spices and herbs to enhance flavor.

Think about canned or frozen varieties: Frozen and canned foods grown from the ground can be a helpful and reasonable choice, particularly when a new product isn't in season.

By eating many fruits and vegetables, we can support our overall health and lower our risk of developing chronic diseases that could result in premature death. Furthermore, an eating routine that is wealthy in products the soil can advance great physical and emotional wellness, which can improve our satisfaction and help us live longer and more satisfying lives.

Controlling one's alcohol intake

Controlling one's alcohol intake is essential to preventing premature death and preserving one's health. While there are some health benefits to drinking moderately, excessive drinking can cause various health issues and raise the risk of chronic diseases. Here are some suggestions for controlling your alcohol intake:

Know what constitutes a beverage: 12 ounces of beer, 5 ounces of wine, or 1.5 ounces of distilled spirits constitute a typical beverage. You can make it easier to track how much alcohol you drink by knowing what constitutes a drink.

Fix limits: Be firm with yourself about your limits. Women should limit themselves to one drink daily for moderate alcohol consumption, while men should limit themselves to two.

Drink water instead of alcoholic beverages: Drinking water between drinks of alcohol can help you stay hydrated and drink less alcohol.

Limit your drinking: Binge drinking, defined as having four or more drinks in two hours for women and five or more drinks in two hours for men, can cause various health issues and increase the likelihood of accidents and injuries.

If you need help, seek assistance from a medical professional or a support group if you struggle to control your alcohol intake. We can support our overall health and lower our risk of developing chronic diseases that could cause premature death by controlling our alcohol consumption. In addition, drinking everyday can improve social interactions and reduce stress, both of which can enhance our quality of life and assist us in living lives that are both longer and more satisfying.

Chapter 2

Exercise regularly

Regular exercise is important for preventing premature death and maintaining good health. Cardiovascular health, the risk of chronic diseases, mental health, and longevity can all be improved through exercise. You can incorporate regular exercise into your life in the following ways:

Choose things you like to do: Find physical activities you enjoy, like swimming, dancing, walking, jogging, cycling, or dancing. This helps you stay motivated and stick to your exercise plan.

Set attainable goals: Goals within your reach include exercising for 30 minutes three to five times per week, for instance. Start with modest objectives and gradually increase your exercise duration and intensity.

Include regular physical activity in your day:

- Walk or bike to work.
- Take the stairs rather than the elevator.
- Walk quickly during your lunch break.

Vary your daily routine: Experiment with various workouts to keep things fresh and push your body. Include exercises for strength training to build muscle and preserve bone density.

Keep your word: Include regular exercise in your routine. Find a workout buddy to help keep you on track or put it on your calendar.

We can support our overall health and lower our risk of developing chronic diseases that could result in premature death by exercising regularly. In addition, regular exercise can improve our mental health, give us more energy, and make us feel better, all of which can improve our quality of life and help us live longer and more satisfying lives.

The significance of the physical activity

Engaging in physical activity is essential to preserving good health and lowering the likelihood of dying too soon. Regular physical activity can have several positive effects on one's health, including:

Worked on cardiovascular well-being: Physical activity regularly can help lower blood pressure, improve heart health, and lower the risk of heart disease and stroke.

Decreased hazard of persistent illnesses: The risk of chronic diseases like type 2 diabetes, obesity, and some types of cancer can all be reduced through physical activity.

Enhanced mental well-being: Physical activity can enhance cognitive function, reduce stress and anxiety, and improve mood.

Extended lifespan: It has been demonstrated that regular physical activity increases longevity and overall quality of life. Adults should participate in muscle-strengthening activities at least two days per week in addition to 150 minutes of moderate-intensity or 75 minutes of vigorous-intensity physical activity per week.

By incorporating regular physical activity into our daily routine, we can support our overall health and lower our risk of developing chronic diseases that could result in premature death. Additionally, physical activity has the potential to enhance our mental and emotional well-being, thereby enhancing our quality of life and enabling us to live lives that are both longer and more satisfying.

The amount of exercise that should be done

The amount of exercise that adults should do is at least 150 minutes of moderate-intensity aerobic physical activity or 75 minutes of vigorous-intensity aerobic physical activity every week. Muscle-strengthening activities should be done at least twice a week.

Activities like brisk walking, cycling, or swimming are examples of moderate-intensity aerobic physical activity, whereas activities like running, aerobic dancing, or playing basketball are examples of vigorous-intensity aerobic physical activity.

Yoga and tai chi, for example, are two examples of activities that can help improve flexibility, balance, and coordination. Before starting a new exercise program, you must talk to a doctor if you're new to exercise or have health issues. Additionally, it is essential to begin with, modest objectives and gradually increase exercise duration and intensity over time.

By exercising the recommended amount, we can support our overall health and lower our risk of developing chronic diseases that could cause premature death. Cardiovascular health, the risk of chronic diseases, mental health, and longevity can all be improved through regular exercise.

Exercises to think about

There are a variety of exercises that can support overall health and lower the risk of dying too soon. Some examples include:

Aerobic activity: Any activity that raises the heart rate and oxygen consumption, such as dancing, brisk walking, running, cycling, or swimming, is considered aerobic exercise. Cardiovascular health can be improved, endurance can be increased, and the risk of chronic diseases like type 2 diabetes and heart disease can be reduced through aerobic exercise.

Strength training: Muscular endurance and strength should be increased. Strength training involves using resistance, like weights or resistance bands. Strength preparation can assist with working on bone thickness, increment bulk, and work by and large actual capability.

Flexibility training: Stretching and yoga are two examples of flexibility exercises that can help improve posture, reduce injury risk, and increase range of motion.

Balance training: Yoga and tai chi are two examples of balance exercises that can aid in maintaining one's equilibrium and lowering one's risk of falling, both of which are crucial for older people.

Because this can assist you in maintaining a regular exercise routine, selecting activities that appeal to you and are compatible with your way of life is essential. In addition, incorporating various exercises can aid in overall fitness enhancement and injury prevention.

Overcoming obstacles to exercise

Several common obstacles to exercise can keep people from exercising the recommended amount. The following are some ways to get around these obstacles:

Time constraint: Particularly for busy people, exercising can be difficult. Schedule exercise into your day, just like you would any other important task, is one strategy. This may assist in making exercise a regular part of your life.

A lack of drive: Staying motivated to exercise can be hard when you're just starting. One option is finding a workout buddy or enrolling in a group fitness class, as social support can boost motivation and accountability.

Inaccessibility to facilities and equipment: Not everyone can access a gym or exercise equipment. In any case, many activities should be possible with practically zero gear, for example, bodyweight activities or strolling outside.

Conditions or bodily injuries: It may be necessary to adapt their exercise routine to accommodate injuries or health conditions. Contacting a medical specialist or trained fitness professional is important when developing a safe and efficient training regimen.

Individuals can increase their likelihood of meeting the recommended amount of physical activity and supporting overall health by identifying and removing common obstacles to exercise. You can also make physical activity a regular and sustainable part of your routine by finding enjoyable and easy activities.

Chapter 3

Avoid High-Risk Behaviors

Engaging in high-risk behaviours can make you more likely to pass away too soon. Avoiding the following high-risk behaviours is recommended:

Smoking: Smoking is linked to numerous health issues, including cancer, heart disease, and stroke, and is a leading cause of preventable death. It can improve overall health and reduce the risk of premature death by quitting smoking.

Excessive drinking of alcohol: Drinking exorbitant measures of liquor can expand the gamble of liver illness, certain tumours, and other medical issues. Moderate alcohol consumption is defined as no more than one drink per day for women and no more than two drinks per day for men.

Using drugs: Using illegal drugs can make you more likely to overdose and have other health issues. If you or someone you know is struggling with addiction, avoiding using drugs and getting help is important.

Drunk driving: Accidents involving motor vehicles and fatalities can be made more likely by reckless driving, such as speeding or driving while under the influence of drugs or alcohol. To reduce the possibility of an accident, it is essential to drive lawfully and responsibly.

Individuals can improve their overall health and reduce their risk of premature death by abstaining from high-risk behaviours. Individuals can also help overcome these behaviours and improve their quality of life by seeking support and treatment for addiction or other health issues.

Giving up smoking

Giving up smoking is one of the most important things a person can do to lower their risk of dying young and improve their overall health. The following are some methods for quitting smoking:

Treatment with nicotine replacement: When quitting smoking, nicotine replacement therapy (NRT) can help alleviate cravings and withdrawal symptoms. NRT comes in patches, gum, and lozenges, among other forms.

Medications: The cravings and withdrawal symptoms associated with quitting smoking can be reduced by taking certain medications, such as bupropion and varenicline. A medical care supplier can endorse these prescriptions.

Behavioural assistance: By providing support, education, and accountability, behavioural support, such as counselling or support groups, can assist individuals in quitting smoking.

Avoid stimuli: Avoiding things like stress and social situations that could encourage smoking is critical. People may be able to maintain their commitment to quitting smoking by recognizing and avoiding these triggers.

Stopping smoking can be testing, yet it is conceivable with the right help and methodologies. By quitting smoking, individuals can improve their overall health and reduce their risk of premature death.

Refraining from using drugs

Refraining from using drugs is an important step that individuals can take to improve their overall health and lower their risk of dying prematurely. Here are a few systems for keeping away from drug use:

Education: People can make better decisions and avoid drug use by being aware of drug risks and consequences.

Taking care of yourself: Peer pressure can have a big impact, especially on young people. It's important to surround yourself with positive people and avoid places where drug use might be common.

Addiction rehabilitation: It is essential to seek assistance from an addiction specialist or healthcare provider if a person is struggling with addiction. Counselling, medication-assisted treatment, or inpatient rehab are all options for treatment.

Managing anxiety: Because stress can lead to drug use, it's important to learn healthy ways to deal with stress, like exercising or meditation.

By abstaining, people can lower their risk of addiction, overdose, and other health issues brought on by drug use. Furthermore, looking for help for fixation can assist people with defeating these ways of behaving and working on their satisfaction.

Safe sex practices

It's important to engage in safe sex practices to cut down on the risk of STIs and other health issues. Safe sex strategies include the following:

Utilize condoms: Correct and consistent use of condoms can help lower the risk of STIs, including HIV.

Take a test: If you're having sex with a new partner, getting tested regularly for STIs is critical.

Restrict sexual partners: Having fewer sexual partners can help lower the risk of sexually transmitted infections (STIs).

Partner with others: Sexually transmitted infections (STIs) can be reduced by openly and honestly discussing sexual health and practices with partners.

People can lower their risk of STIs and other health issues linked to sexual activity by engaging in safe sex practices. In addition, obtaining STI testing and treatment can assist individuals in overcoming these health issues and enhancing their quality of life.

Chapter 4
Get Enough Sleep

Sleeping enough is important for your health and well-being as a whole. Some methods for getting enough sleep are as follows:

Establish a routine for your sleep: The body's internal clock can be regulated, and sleep quality can be improved by going to bed and getting up at the same time every day.

Make a peaceful sleeping environment: Promoting sleep can be made easier by establishing a cool, dark bedroom that is comfortable and conducive to sleep.

Cut back on alcohol and caffeine: Caffeine and liquor can obstruct rest, so it is vital to restrict utilization, especially before sleep time.

Avoid using a screen before bed: Electronic devices' blue light can disrupt sleep, so it's important to avoid using them before bedtime.

People can lower their risk of heart disease, diabetes, and obesity—all linked to sleep deprivation—by getting enough sleep. A good night's sleep can also help with mood, concentration, and overall quality of life.

The importance of getting enough sleep for good health

Sleep is essential for good health in general. It's important to get enough sleep for the following reasons:

Physical fitness: Sleep is essential to physical health because it allows the body to repair and reenergize itself. It is related to a diminished gamble of medical conditions, like coronary illness, diabetes, and heftiness.

Mental wellness: Sleep can improve mood, reduce stress, and improve cognitive function, all of which are important for mental health.

Immune system: Sleep is essential for immune function because it enables the body to produce and distribute immune cells and cytokines, which aid in the fight against infection and inflammation.

Safety: Sleep deprivation can make it harder to think clearly and make accidents and injuries more likely.

By getting enough sleep, people can improve their mental and physical health, boost their immune systems, and lower their risk of accidents and injuries. Also, getting enough sleep can make life better in general.

The amount of sleep that is recommended

The recommended amount of sleep can vary based on an individual's age and requirements. The general recommendations for various age groups are as follows:

Infants aged 0 to 3 months 14 to 17 hours' daily

Infants (4 to 11 months): 12 to 15 hours a day

Toddlers (under a year): 11 to 14 hours per day

Preschoolers (ages 3-5): 10-13 hours out of every day

School-matured kids (6-13 years) and Teenagers between the ages of 14 and 17: 8 to 10 hours per day

Adults (age 18 to 64): 7-9 hours per day

Seniors Adults (65 and older): 7 to 8 hours a day

It's important to remember that people's sleep requirements can vary based on things like genetics, lifestyle, and health conditions. To support your overall health and well-being, listening to your body and placing a high value on getting enough sleep is essential.

Ways to improve the quality of your sleep

Here are some ways to improve the quality of your sleep: Establish a routine for your sleep: The body's internal clock can be regulated, and sleep quality can be improved by going to bed and getting up at the same time every day.

Make a peaceful sleeping environment: Promoting sleep can be made easier by establishing a cool, dark bedroom that is comfortable and conducive to sleep.

Cut back on alcohol and caffeine: Caffeine and alcohol can make sleeping hard, so it's important to cut back, especially before bed.

Avoid using a screen before bed: Electronic devices' blue light can disrupt sleep, so it's important to avoid using them before bedtime.

Relaxation techniques to try: Meditation, deep breathing and progressive muscle relaxation are all forms of relaxation that can assist in promoting relaxation and enhancing the quality of one's sleep.

Regular exercise: Regular exercise can improve the quality of your sleep, but it's important not to do it too close to bedtime.

Do not nap: Even though it can be tempting to nap, it can disrupt sleep at night, so it is important to avoid napping or limit naps to 30 minutes.

People can improve the quality of their sleep and their overall health and well-being by putting these methods into practice. Talking to a doctor about any underlying health issues that might prevent you from sleeping is crucial if your sleep problems don't disappear.

Chapter 5

How to Manage Stress

Stress is a normal part of life, but too much stress can harm your mental and physical health. Here are some ways to deal with stress:

Determine the cause of your stress: People can take steps to address the underlying cause of stress by determining the source.

Relaxation techniques: Relaxation methods like yoga, deep breathing, or meditation can help people relax and feel less stressed.

Regular exercise: Regular exercise has been shown to improve mood, well-being, and stress levels.

Give self-care priority: Stress levels can be reduced by participating in self-care activities like getting enough sleep, eating a healthy diet, and having fun.

Seek assistance: People can learn effective coping mechanisms and cope with stress by talking to friends, family, or a mental health professional.

Effective time management: Putting tasks in order of importance and breaking them down into smaller, more manageable steps can reduce stress and increase productivity. By implementing these strategies, people can effectively manage their stress levels and improve their overall health and well-being. If stress levels overwhelm or interfere with daily activities, getting help is important.

Health effects of stress

Excessive or persistent stress can negatively affect mental and physical health. The health effects of stress include the following:

Heart disease is more likely: Blood pressure, cholesterol levels, and inflammation can all rise due to chronic stress, which can also increase the risk of heart disease.

Insufficient immune system: Stress can weaken the immune system, making people more likely to get sick and get sicker.

Gastrointestinal issues: Digestive issues like indigestion, stomach pain, and diarrhea can be brought on by stress.

Issues with mental health: Anxiety and depression are two mental health issues that can be exacerbated by chronic stress.

Sleep issues: Sleep problems like insomnia and other sleep disorders can be brought on by stress.

Skin issues: Acne, eczema, and psoriasis are skin conditions caused by chronic stress.

It is essential to recognize stress's potential health effects and effectively manage stress levels. Individuals can reduce the negative effects of stress on health and improve their overall well-being by implementing strategies for stress management and seeking support when needed.

Strategies for stress management

Numerous strategies can assist individuals in effectively managing stress. Some examples include:

Meditation in mindfulness: The practice of mindfulness meditation entails paying attention to the now without judging. It may aid in stress reduction and overall well-being enhancement.

Progressive muscle relaxation includes tensing and relaxing different bodily muscle groups to encourage relaxation and lessen stress levels.

Breathing deeply: To promote relaxation and lower stress levels, deep breathing exercises involve taking slow, deep breaths.

Yoga helps people relax and feel less stressed by incorporating meditation, breathing exercises, and physical postures.

Exercise: Regular exercise has been shown to improve mood, well-being, and stress levels.

Management of time: Putting tasks in order of importance and breaking them down into smaller, more manageable steps can reduce stress and increase productivity.

Social assistance: People can learn effective coping mechanisms and cope with stress by talking to friends, family, or a mental health professional.

It is crucial to find methods that work best for each person and incorporate them into daily life. People can improve their health and well-being by effectively managing their stress levels.

Developing resilience to stress

Resilience is the capacity to effectively deal with and adapt to stressful circumstances. The following are some methods that can assist individuals in developing resilience to stress:

Maintain a positive attitude: People who cultivate a positive outlook can become more resilient to stress.

Learn how to solve problems: People can feel more in control and better prepared to handle stressful situations by learning how to solve problems.

Obtain support from others: During stressful times, strong social connections can be a source of emotional support.

Make time for yourself: Self-care practices like getting enough sleep, maintaining a healthy diet, and engaging in enjoyable activities can help people become more resilient to stress.

Get professional assistance: Individuals can receive tools and strategies for coping with stress and developing resilience by speaking with a mental health professional.

Put stress-management strategies into practice: Stress-management techniques like yoga, deep breathing, or mindfulness meditation can help you become more resilient. Resilience to stress can be developed over time with effort and dedication. By implementing these strategies, people can improve their overall health and well-being and build resilience to stress.

Chapter 6

Keep Up with Your Medical Checkups

Regular medical checkups are important for keeping your health good and preventing serious health issues. Important reasons to keep up with medical checkups include the following:

Problems with one's health can be found early: Health issues can be detected earlier, when they are easier to treat and manage, with regular checkups.

Keeping an eye on chronic conditions: To keep an eye on chronic conditions and ensure that they are being managed effectively, regular checkups are necessary.

Detection of diseases: Screening tests for diabetes, high blood pressure, and cancer may be part of a medical checkup.

Keeping up vaccinations: People's immunization status can be checked regularly, which can help stop infectious diseases from spreading.

Assessment of health in general: An individual's overall health can be evaluated, and recommendations for health improvement or maintenance are made during a medical checkup.

Based on their age, sex, and overall health, people need to schedule regular medical checkups with their healthcare providers. This can assist in ensuring that any health issues are identified and treated promptly, and that overall health and well-being are maintained.

The significance of getting checked out regularly

Regular checking out is essential for preserving good health and avoiding serious health issues. Important reasons to keep up with medical checkups include the following:

Problems with one's health can be found early: Health issues can be detected earlier, when they are easier to treat and manage, with regular checkups. This may increase the likelihood of successful treatment and improve health outcomes.

Keeping diseases at bay: Screening tests for diseases like diabetes, high blood pressure, and cancer may be included in routine exams. These tests can assist in determining risk factors and preventing disease before its onset.

Controlling chronic conditions: Regular checkups are necessary to keep an eye on chronic conditions and ensure they are being managed effectively. This can assist with forestalling entanglements and work on personal satisfaction.

Health care for the whole person: Clinical checkups open the door to medical services suppliers to survey a singular's general well-being and give suggestions for improving or keeping up with well-being. This may include advice on diet, exercise, and other aspects of one's lifestyle.

A sense of calm: Having peace of mind knowing that any potential health issues are being monitored and addressed can be provided by regular medical examinations.

Based on their age, sex, and overall health, people need to schedule regular medical checkups with their healthcare providers. This can assist in ensuring that any health issues are identified and treated promptly, and that overall health and well-being are maintained.

Considerable tests and screenings

The specific tests and screenings suggested during a medical checkup can vary based on age, sex, family history, and overall health. However, the following are some typical examinations and screenings that healthcare professionals might suggest:

Tension in the body: A blood pressure test determines the force that the blood exerts against the arteries' walls. Heart disease and stroke are more likely in people with high blood pressure.

Cholesterol: The levels of various cholesterols in the blood are determined by a cholesterol test. Heart disease risk can rise when "bad" cholesterol (LDL) levels are high.

Blood sugar: A blood glucose test estimates how much glucose (sugar) is in the blood. Diabetes can be diagnosed by having high blood glucose levels.

Cancer examinations: Screenings for cancers like breast, cervical, prostate, colon, and lung may be recommended by healthcare providers based on age, sex, and other factors.

Immunizations: Immunizations against infectious diseases like shingles, influenza, and pneumonia may be recommended by healthcare providers.

Pap test: A Pap smear is a test that is done on women to check for cervical cancer.

Mammogram: A mammogram is an X-ray to screen women for breast cancer.

A healthcare provider can advise on the most appropriate tests based on a person's specific health history and risk factors, so it's important to talk to them about any concerns or questions about recommended tests and screenings.

Conclusion

In conclusion, living a long and fulfilling life necessitates avoiding premature death and maintaining good health. Individuals can increase their chances of staying healthy and avoiding serious health problems by adhering to general principles like eating a healthy diet, exercising regularly, avoiding high-risk behaviours, getting enough sleep, managing stress, and keeping up with medical checkups. It is essential to prioritise self-care and incorporate healthy choices into daily life. By doing this, people can improve their quality of life and lower their risk of dying too soon or developing serious health issues.

Recap of important hints for avoiding premature death

Yes, the following are important hints for avoiding premature death:

Eat a well-balanced diet, avoid processed and high-sugar foods, eat many fruits and vegetables, and drink moderately to maintain a healthy diet.

At least 150 minutes of physical activity per week, including both cardio and strength training, is required for regular exercise.

Smoking, drug use, and inappropriate sex are all high-risk behaviours to avoid.

Set a regular sleep schedule, create a relaxing environment, and aim for 7-9 hours per night to get enough sleep.

Build resilience and manage stress using yoga, deep breathing, and meditation.

Get the recommended tests and screenings based on age, sex, and health history to keep up with your medical checkups.

People can improve their overall health and well-being by incorporating these suggestions into their daily lives, lowering their risk of dying too soon or developing serious health issues.

A push to put health and wellness first

I'd be happy to encourage you to put health and wellness first!

One of the most important things a person can do is take care of their health. People can improve their quality of life, spend more time with loved ones, and lower their risk of developing serious health issues by prioritising health and wellness.

It can be hard to make healthy choices in a busy and fast-paced world, but it's important to remember that even small changes can make a big difference. It can improve one's health and well-being by making even insignificant adjustments, such as walking during one's lunch break, selecting healthier foods, and getting enough sleep.

Additionally, it is essential to remember that self-care is not selfish. Individuals can better care for others and positively impact their communities if they take care of themselves.

As a result, I urge you to place your health and well-being first and to make small changes each day to boost your overall health. You can live a long, happy, and fulfilling life by investing in your health. You deserve to feel your best.